Renal Diet HQ IQ
Teaching You To Master Your Health

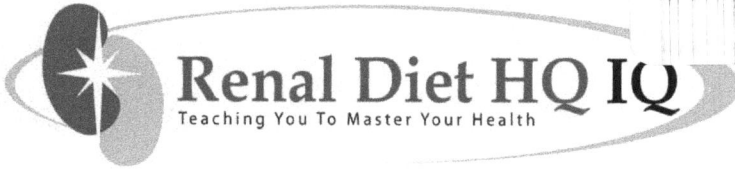

Sexuality and Chronic Kidney Disease For Men and Women: A Path To Better Understanding

Book 10

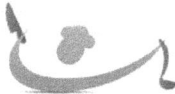

RENALDIET
HEADQUARTERS
BY HEALTHY DIET MENUS FOR YOU

Purpose and Introduction

What I have found through the emails and requests of my readers is that it is difficult to find information about a pre-dialysis kidney lifestyle that is actionable. I want you to know that is what I intend to provide in all my books.

I wrote this book with you in mind: the person with kidney problems who does not know where to start or can't seem to get the answers that you need from other sources. This book will provide information that is applicable to a predialysis kidney disease lifestyle.

Who am I? I am a registered dietitian in the USA who has been working with kidney patients for my entire 15 + years of experience. Find all my books on Amazon on my author page: http://www.amazon.com/Mathea-Ford/e/B008E1E7IS/

My goals are simple – to give some answers and to create an understanding of what is typical. In this series of 12 books, I will take you through the different parts of being a person with pre-dialysis kidney disease. It will not necessarily be what happens in your case, as everyone is an individual. I may simplify things in an effort to write them so that I feel you can learn the most from the information. This may mean that I don't say the exact things that your doctor would say. If you don't understand, please ask your doctor.

I want you to know, I am not a medical doctor and I am not aware of your particular condition. Information in this book is current as of publication, but may or may not have changed. This book is not meant to substitute for medical treatment for you, your friends, your caregivers, or your family members. You should not base treatment decisions solely on what is contained in this book. Develop your treatment plan with your doctors, nurses and the other medical professionals on your team. I recommend that you double-check any information with your medical team to verify if it applies to you.

In other words, I am not responsible for your medical care. I am providing this book for information and entertainment purposes, not medical diagnoses. Please consult with your doctor about any questions that you have about your particular case.

Table of Contents

Introduction

Chronic kidney disease (CKD) can have many effects on the body when it comes to physical symptoms, but one of its biggest tolls is widely overlooked and shouldn't be ignored: sexuality. Many people diagnosed with chronic kidney disease notice a difference in numerous aspects of their sexuality.

Sexuality includes not only sexual health, but also the way individuals feel about their body and how they communicate and relate to their partners. There are lots of reasons why these things might be affected. For instance, chronic kidney disease (CKD) can cause chemical changes in the body that affect circulation, nerve function, hormones and energy levels. In addition, any underlying health conditions that contribute to CKD such as high blood pressure or diabetes might also affect sexuality as well.

Some of the symptoms associated with CKD, such as fatigue, can lead to a loss of interest in sexual activity. Other physical symptoms can make it difficult to reach orgasm while emotional problems that can accompany chronic illnesses, such as depression and anxiety, can cause their own sexual side effects.

Luckily, with some of the recent advances in the medical management of CKD, such as dialysis and transplantation, the well-being and lifestyles of those with kidney disease have significantly improved. This means that there has also been an improvement in the sexual health and function of those living with CKD. Still, maintaining a healthy and gratifying sex life and rewarding relationship in regards to your sexuality can be challenging at times.

Your sexuality is an important part of who you are as an individual and is an essential part of how you communicate within your relationship. It is far more than simply about sexual intercourse. It involves how you identify yourself in regards to your gender, the giving and receiving of pleasure, and the desire for intimacy. The good news is, even with the issues that CKD can impose, medical interventions, different kinds of therapies, and relationship counseling are available to help manage the effects of CKD in order to improve this area of your life so that it can be fulfilling and enjoyable again.

With proper communication between you, your partner, and your medical team, many of these issues can be overcome and are treatable. In the following book we'll discuss some of the common problems that chronic kidney disease patients face when it comes to their sexuality and how these issues might be treated and conquered.

Why Your Sexuality Is Important

Sexuality can be an awkward topic to talk about, even in a medical sense and it's not usually a topic that gets discussed. It's a subject that can bring on a range of emotions and feelings since it is so closely entwined with intimacy. For those with a chronic illness, it can bring up many feelings, including guilt, inadequacy, sadness, and even fear. Although there might still be moments of pleasure, most of the time it probably feels as though those are still too few and far between as you're worrying about feeling too tired, stressed, or overwhelmed with everything else going on.

Think about it, ever since you have been old enough to say the word, people have been "shushing" you to be quiet. It's something to be kept to yourself, and not discussed out loud. Perhaps you grew up in an era where pregnancy was not even mentioned on TV! They show lots more on TV now, but it's still something that personally you probably would prefer not to talk about. It's an awkward subject, and talking about it to your doctor seems like a bother to him or her, right? Have you prescribed to the myth that it's just not important? Or that your needs are not that important? Or maybe you are thinking about the fact that you will see that doctor again next month, and it will be embarrassing for you. [Never mind that he or she sees lots of people between now and then and they also talk to people about lots of things – much more delicate than this!] The fact of the matter is that if you are concerned about sex or sexuality, you should discuss it so you can see if there is a cause and a solution. Normalizing this part of your life is important.

Still, sexuality is a very important element for our overall happiness and for a satisfying partnership. Studies have discovered that fulfilled partners see sexual activity as one of their many sources of pleasure and intimacy. On the other hand, unhappy partners focus on sexual activity and frequently view it as one of the main causes of their problems.

Sex can often be the first thing that affects a relationship when it breaks down, though it's not always the *primary* problem. Sexual activity is partly based on how a couple connects with one another and when they no longer connect in that way, they are losing a major part of their intimacy. When the sex becomes obsolete, they start losing one of their strongest bonds with one another.

One of the major reasons that sexual activity, and by "sexual activity" we're not just referring to intercourse, is so important to a relationship is because it's one of the few parameters in a partnership that differentiates your relationship from others. When that element is no longer as prevalent then it can be more difficult to define the boundaries of the partnership and set it apart from other relationships in your life. This can lead to feelings of confusion and frustration for both partners. It can also lead to loss of connectedness. For the individual with the chronic kidney disease, it can be challenging to work through the physical problems that make sexual activity difficult. For the partner, it can be challenging to work through the emotions that come along with feeling frustrated and oftentimes helpless in a situation that they have seemingly little control over.

Learning to redefine your sexuality within your relationship is important when you are dealing with a chronic medical condition. You might have to readjust your way of thinking. Although you can still have a healthy, passionate, and secure relationship, you might have to realize that the foundation is built on something more than quantity of sexual acts. This could mean learning to forgive yourself for not living up to the person you were in the past and acknowledging the fact that while the goals you might reach in the future might seem small, they are still worthwhile.

Suggestions for Redefining Your Sexuality with CKD

- Keep in mind that although you're still a sexual person you may need to explore new ways to enjoy your sexuality.
- Focus on pleasure instead of performance.
- Don't worry so much about the destination. This time, it really *is* about the journey.
- Communicate with your partner about how you're feeling. What might feel like an awkward conversation might help you feel more comfortable in the bedroom now.
- Don't be afraid to ask for what you want.
- Explore new ways of doing things and don't forget to laugh if they don't work. If you can't laugh with your partner then it's almost impossible to do anything else with them.
- Remember there are many pleasurable and satisfying sexual activities that do not involve intercourse.
- Read books and watch movies to get new ideas.
- Don't underestimate the power of vaginal dryness if you are a woman. Many sexual problems are caused by dryness and are easily solved with a lubricant.
- Plan for sexual activity during times when you don't have anything else going on and can give it your full attention.

Effects On Sexuality

Your CKD can have a variety of different effects on your sexuality. Where you were once sexually active, for various reasons, you find that your interest in sexual activity wanes or that you are unable to engage in intercourse as you once were. As someone who was once able to enjoy intercourse, this can be disheartening and frustrating for both you and your partner and have an undesirable effect on your relationship.

A lot of people only think that sexuality only refers to the act of intercourse itself. In actuality, it really includes numerous aspects, such as how individuals communicate with their partners and even how they feel about their own inner level of confidence. Sexuality also involves a variety of enjoyable activities of a sexual nature that may or may not include intercourse or penetration.

Is Sexual Intercourse Safe?

One of the first questions that cross many people's minds is whether or not sexual intercourse is actually safe for the individual with CKD. It's true that there are some patients with chronic illnesses who must avoid certain sexual activities, especially activities that might increase their heart rates to unhealthy levels. Some individuals and their partners are concerned that sexual intercourse might damage the dialysis access or transplanted kidney. However, no sexual limitations really need to be placed on chronic kidney disease patients. As long as sexual activity doesn't place pressure on the vascular access site, it won't cause any damage. Most individuals find that they are able to have normal, healthy sexual relations even when they are undergoing dialysis, as long as they are mindful of their access site.

When Intercourse Is Not Possible

There might be times when intercourse is not possible. This could happen for a variety of reasons, most of which will be discussed later at length. During the times when sexual intercourse is not possible, either for physical or emotional reasons, there are still ways that intimacy can be achieved. It does not have to be avoided altogether. Activities such as snuggling, hugging, and kissing can provide feelings of warmth and closeness even if the actual act of intercourse is not involved.

For most couples, the feeling of intimacy that comes with having an emotional relationship is just as important as the aspects of having a physical relationship. This feeling of intimacy is closely tied in with the physical aspects of sexual activity. Sometimes, however, changes might occur that call for a need to alter your physical relationship. During alterations in medication or other periods when there are changes in your partner's libido there might be a need to adjust your physical relationship.

Losing Desire To Be Sexually Active

At some point during the course of living with chronic kidney disease you might find that you lose the desire to be sexually active. There are many reasons why this might occur and it's not uncommon. Use of certain medications, may cause weight gain, acne, and unwanted hair growth or loss which could cause body image problems. Surgical scars can cause some individuals to feel unattractive. Medical changes and changes in self-image may affect sexual interest and functioning.

Chronic kidney disease can cause physical and emotional changes that may have an effect on your sex life. For instance, the chemical changes that occur in the body with kidney disease can influence hormones, circulation, nerve function, and energy levels. As a result, these changes more often than not lower sexual interest and can even lower sexual ability. When this happens, you might not lose interest in sexual activity but be physically unable to perform. As a result, over time, you might lose interest in sexual activity simply because your body is unable to perform and your mind finds this frustrating. In addition, physical changes may cause those with chronic kidney disease to feel less attractive which can affect them sexually.

The following is a list of additional reasons that may have an effect on the libido.

- **Medications:** Some medications, especially those used to treat blood pressure and depression, have sexual side effects. They can make sexual arousal difficult and many individuals notice a decrease in their sex drive. Some medications also have weight gain as a side effect which can lead to body image issues.
- **Depression:** Depression can lead to a lack of interest in activities that individuals once held an interest in. Depression can also make sexual arousal more difficult and lead to an inability to reach orgasm easily.
- **Fatigue:** Fatigue is one of the most common symptoms of kidney disease. A kidney-friendly diet or meal plan designed to limit the amount of waste that can build up in your body can help with fatigue. Individuals with end stage renal disease may feel tired after their dialysis. Ongoing fatigue should be discussed with your doctor.
- **Sleep disorders:** Lack of sleep can lead to fatigue. Tiredness can cause weakness and a decrease in sexual activity. Sleep apnea is very common for those who have CKD and results in a disruption in breathing during sleep. For some, during a deep sleep breathing can stop for as long as 10 seconds. Obstruction and snoring can cause the individual to wake up

frequently throughout the night. This can lead to restless sleep which can cause tiredness throughout the day.

- **Hypertension:** High blood pressure can lead to erectile dysfunction in men. In women, it can cause vaginal dryness and pain during intercourse.
- **Physical discomfort:** Pain, dryness, and other physical discomfort can make sexual intercourse and even arousal uncomfortable. As a result, the idea of intercourse or sexual activity at all can be off-putting for some individuals.
- **Anxiety:** Anxiety can cause stress and tension which can create difficulties with arousal and reaching orgasm. Anxiety can manifest from stress relating to medical problems or about other issues surrounding your CKD. Sometimes anxiety can also be a side effect of medications.
- **Uremia (extra waste in the blood):** High levels of wastes or toxins may cause low energy levels, nausea, poor memory, and difficulty concentrating. These can affect your interest in sexual activity. Making changes to your diet and dialysis can reduce toxin build-up and help you feel better.
- **Anemia:** Anemia can cause fatigue and weakness, making it difficult to find the energy to enjoy sexual intercourse or to participate in any sexual activity.
- **Leg cramps:** Leg cramps can cause restless leg syndrome, leading to insomnia which can make sleeping difficult. As a result, the individual may feel tired and weak during the day and sore and painful at night.
- **Excess Fluid**: A lot of people undergoing dialysis treatment must limit their fluid intake. You'll probably feel unwell if there is excess fluid in your body since your blood pressure will rise, and your heart must work harder. You'll be breathless, and you'll be bloated. You will probably have less energy as well and these symptoms can cause a lack of sexual interest.

- **Hormones:** Different hormones control and influence sexual interest and fertility. CKD can affect hormone levels and you may have noticed the effects of these changes such as a change in libido and sexual function. Menstrual periods may become irregular or stop and men may experience erectile difficulties, reduced sperm counts, and motility.
- **Neuropathy**: Nerve damage or neuropathy can occur in those who have CKD. If the genital area is affected then it could cause pain, making sexual intercourse uncomfortable.
- **Vitamin and Trace Metal Depletion**: Vitamins and trace minerals can be depleted during dialysis. The depletion of zinc during this process could lead to sexual dysfunction. Discuss with your doctor any necessary laboratory testing for vitamin and mineral levels to determine deficiencies.

Female Sexuality

Generally speaking, women tend to experience sexual issues slightly more frequently than men when it comes to chronic illnesses. The *Collaborative Depression and Sexual Dysfunction in Hemodialysis Working Group* conducted a study and examined the responses of 659 female dialysis patients in Europe and South America who completed a questionnaire called the Female Sexual Function Index. The findings discovered that 84% of all women and 55% of sexually active women in the study experienced sexual problems. Of the women surveyed, those with a partner were less likely to report sexual dysfunction than those without a partner.

In addition, sexual dysfunction occurred more frequently in women who were older, less educated, had symptoms of depression, had diabetes, had reached menopause, and took diuretics. Almost all the women (96%) who weren't on a waiting list for transplants and were living without a partner reported sexual dysfunction.

Sometimes a decreased interest in sexual activity occurs without any explanation at all. This can lead to feelings of guilt and frustration. Most of the time, however, it can be explained by taking a look at your medical history-either through your physical or emotional symptoms. The important thing to consider is whether or not you're actually experiencing a decreased interest in sexual activity, having pain with intercourse, or if you are unable to reach orgasm, which are three different issues but all plague those with CKD.

Lower hormone levels, for instance, may cause some women to experience vaginal dryness or painful intercourse. Some medications cause hormonal changes making it hard for a woman to become sexually aroused or achieve an orgasm. In addition, the side effects of some medicines and complications from uremia can lead to fatigue, menstrual irregularities, and a decrease in sexual desire.

Anemia can be treated but in some cases, it's difficult to determine what the underlying cause of the problem is.

Body Image Issues

Some women might experience a decline in their libido due to body image issues. Since sexual activity is based, in large part, on emotional connections, if women aren't completely in tune with themselves, they often have difficulty connecting sexually. Chronic kidney disease can have physical ramifications on a woman's body which, in turn, can have effects on a woman's libido. Some women might find that they gain weight, lose weight, get stretch marks, lose their hair, or have other physical changes that make them feel unattractive. A catheter in the stomach or fistula in the arm may also create anxiety either because a woman is afraid it's unattractive or is worried it might be damaged.

As a result, they might have trouble getting interested in being intimate with their partner due to lack of self-confidence. If you have these feelings, then it's important to share them with your partner. Sharing them is usually the best way to conquer them.

Depression: Decreased Interest in Sexual Activity

Sometimes women experience a decreased interest in sexual activity without any reason at all, but this is rare. More often than not, it can be chalked up to either a medication issue, which can normally be fixed by changing medications or dosages, or a hormonal change. In some instances, it is depression or anxiety.

Symptoms of depression include:

- Trouble concentrating and making decisions
- Fatigue and lack of energy
- Feelings of remorse, worthlessness, or helplessness

- Feelings of despair
- Insomnia or sleeping too much
- Anxiety
- Agitation
- Loss of interest in activities you once enjoyed
- Eating too much or loss of appetite
- Constant aches and pains, headaches, or digestive problems that don't go away
- Constant distressing, worried, or "empty" feelings
- Suicidal thoughts/attempts of suicide

If this occurs, it is very important to talk to your doctor because there are other symptoms that are more than likely accompanying the distress and it's imperative that you get this addressed. Depression is not usually something that merely "goes away" on its own and is something that must be treated. It is also something that is not uncommon when being diagnosed.

According to the National Institute of Mental Health, 19 million American adults struggle with depression at some point. The rate of depression is even higher for those who are diagnosed with chronic illnesses. It is possible that as many as 40% of the individuals with CKD will experience some form of depression after diagnosis. Not all forms of depression are chronic, but all symptoms should be talked about with your doctor, especially if you that they're not relieved after a couple of weeks on their own.

Difficulty In Achieving Orgasm

The initial interest in sexual activity might be present, but you might have trouble achieving orgasm which can also lead to feelings of frustration. Officially referred to as "orgasmic dysfunction", most likely it is a hormonal change, especially if you are undergoing dialysis or if menstruation has stopped altogether. Certain medications might also make reaching orgasm more difficult. If you are not undergoing dialysis, then extra stimulation might be needed for orgasm.

First, it must be determined whether the issue is physical, hormonal, or emotional. Treatment can involve such things as education, cognitive behavioral therapy, and teaching orgasm by focusing on pleasurable stimulation (mainly beneficial to those who have had difficulty achieving orgasm even before the diagnosis of CKD). Certain medical problems, new medications, or untreated depression are evaluated and treated for orgasmic dysfunction to improve, too, if emotional issues are not discovered. If there are additional sexual dysfunctions present, such as lack of interest and pain, then these are usually addressed as part of the treatment plan as well.

Pain with Intercourse

Pain with intercourse, which might not have been present in the past, might make sexual activity uncomfortable. This could be due to medications which might cause dryness. If this is the case, then talking to your doctor could be helpful. Changing medications or using lubricant for the dryness could be an easy solution for this problem.

In some cases, however, the problem might actually be psychological. Sometimes, anxiety and stress can cause the pelvic muscles to involuntarily clench. Learning stress relieving techniques can be helpful if this is what is going on. Couples therapy or counseling is one way of alleviating these issues, as is opening the doors of communication to get to any underlying problems that might be triggering the response. Sometimes it can take several attempts at treatments, either through counseling or anti-anxiety medication, before a remedy is found since it's not always easy to determine the underlying cause.

Menopause

Dialysis helps to remove wastes from the blood when kidney failure occurs, though it doesn't replace all the kidneys' functions. Dialysis, for instance, doesn't produce hormones. As a result, there are some precautions that menopausal women are suggested to take, especially those who are on dialysis.

Generally speaking, menopausal women are encouraged to take calcium in order to avoid osteoporosis. Women on dialysis or who have a kidney transplant usually have their calcium levels tested to ensure that they're at healthy levels so that they are neither too low nor too high. In menopause, when hormone production decreases it puts women at risk for osteoporosis and heart disease. Since a lot of women on dialysis usually don't have regular periods, they may already have compromised hormone levels. Additional calcium in your diet can help you keep bone loss from occurring as long as your doctor approves.

An increased risk for heart disease is also at stake for menopausal women because of the lower hormone levels. If you have a hysterectomy then you'll have early onset menopause which will put you at risk even sooner. It's therefore important to talk to your doctor about your cardiovascular and bone health early on since it can affect those with CKD more often.

Lastly, lower hormone levels can create vaginal dryness and sometimes even an increased risk of yeast infections. Using a lubricant and talking to your doctor about medications to clear up infections will help keep your pelvic area healthy and safe.

The best thing you can do is educate yourself about these issues now so that you can be aware. This will help you feel comfortable about these issues so you can discuss them with your doctors later. It's also important to know that you are definitely not alone in this journey.

Male Sexuality

Although men might also suffer from similar issues regarding sexuality, some of their difficulties might be different.

Men with kidney failure commonly have issues concerning a lack of desire for sex, erectile dysfunction, or decreased levels of testosterone. Although it can be difficult for most men to talk about their sexuality, your physician or social worker is trained to listen and offer advice or referrals to other professionals. You may even want to consider couples counseling together with a licensed therapist, depending on the situation.

The following is a short list of some of the problems that men with chronic kidney disease might face in regards to their sexuality.

Erectile Dysfunction

Erectile dysfunction (ED) is commonly referred to as "impotence" and affects many men, even those who don't have chronic kidney disease. An estimated 20-30 million men in the United States have problems with impotence. It can occur when blood vessels and nerves to the penis become injured. If the penis doesn't have proper blood flow, it can't maintain an erection.

Diabetes and high blood pressure, the leading causes of chronic kidney disease, are both conditions that can affect blood flow and weaken the blood vessels. Occasionally, ED is a side effect of certain medications, especially those that are taken to control blood pressure. It is important to talk to your doctor about any medications that you are taking if you experience impotence because these might be changed to something else. Other causes of ED can include:

- changes in hormone levels

- build up of waste and fluid in the blood
- problems with blood circulation
- nerve damage
- anemia
- low vitamin and trace metal levels, e.g. zinc
- reduced strength and energy levels
- low self-esteem
- body image problems
- depression, anxiety and stress
- fear of being unable to perform sexually

Psychological Effects

Sometimes stress and anxiety can have psychological effects on sexuality and can lead to difficulty achieving ejaculation, if not arousal. A man might be able to become sexually aroused, for instance, but not be able to reach ejaculation. This can be frustrating and embarrassing and make him unwilling to be involved in future sexual encounters for fear of rejection from his partner. Delayed ejaculation or failure to ejaculate should be discussed with your physician since stress and anxiety could continue to intensify the problem and turn it into a vicious cycle.

Worry and stress can both be parts of CKD and have impacts on sexuality. You might feel worried, nervous, or depressed when faced with chronic kidney disease or kidney failure. Although the feelings are normal, they might cause a loss of energy and lower interest in activities that you used to enjoy, like sex. Worrying about how chronic kidney disease may affect your employment and your family life can also affect your sex life.

The feelings that can accompany CKD can be overpowering. If you feel as though they are overwhelming, it's important to talk to your physician. It's especially important to talk to your doctor or social worker right away if you start having feelings of anxiety or depression.

Body Image Issues

Although body image issues are normally something associated with women, many men feel they may be less attractive due to the physical changes related to their condition or treatment. Individuals with chronic kidney disease sometimes experience undesirable changes to their bodies. Some symptoms like weight gain or loss, breath and body odor, complexion issues, or unusual facial or body hair may occur. A man on dialysis may feel uncomfortable about how his vascular access site appears. Men on peritoneal dialysis may worry about the appearance of their abdomens. These issues might give you body image problems which could make sexual performances awkward and difficult where there weren't issues in the past.

You should always discuss any uncomfortable changes with your partner and healthcare team. Some physical changes are only temporary, while others may point toward a health complication that needs immediate attention.

Fear of Rejection

Due to their medical conditions and any complications they might be facing, some men might feel as though they are not as vigorous as they used to be and are therefore not as "complete." They might have a fear of rejection which might make it difficult for them to approach intimacy as they once did. They might also have a fear of rejection for not appearing as healthy and young as they used to, either to their partners or to potential partners. Vitality is important to many men and having a serious medical condition might feel limiting even if it doesn't actually limit them in a physical sense from the things that they enjoy doing.

Loss of Interest/Hormonal Changes

Women are often the ones who are associated with having hormonal problems when it comes to having low sex drives but men can also have hormonal issues as well.

Hormones are chemicals that are produced by the body's endocrine system. The endocrine system is complicated group of hormone-producing glands that is located throughout the body. The glands help control almost everything from growth to sexual development. In women, estrogens, which generate estradiol, are responsible for the libido. Both men and women have androgens. They produce testosterone and are associated with male levels of sexual arousal.

The kidneys are part of the endocrine system. The adrenal glands, which are located at the top of the kidneys, produce certain hormones. Some men with renal disease might discover that they have hormone levels which become out of balance, thus giving them a loss of interest in sexual activity when this wasn't a problem for them in the past.

If hormones are the issues then your physician will be able to tell a difference in your hormone levels by carrying out some simple blood work. Medication may be used to rectify the problem.

Body Image Issues

Although body image issues have been mentioned, it's important to talk about them in-depth. A lot of individuals end up frustrated with bodies that, at times, can feel as though you have no control over.

A lot of the medications that are taken along with CKD can cause side effects that can lead to body image problems. Some of these side effects can include skin rashes, weight loss, hair loss or thinning, swelling, weight gain, and pale complexions. Sudden weight loss may result in loose skin while weight gain may result in stretch marks.

Additional body changes that can occur with CKD include:

- body odor
- bruising
- decreased endurance and energy levels
- extra fluid from fluid retention or carrying dialysis fluid
- hair loss or gain
- bad breath or a 'coated' tongue
- reduced ability or inability to reach orgasm
- skin changes such as itchiness, dryness or color
- strength and control
- weight changes

How to Feel Good About Yourself

So, how can you avoid body image issues and continue enjoying your sexuality and feeling good about yourself?

Exercise –Physical activity is very important. Although it might be difficult, it's essential if you want to stay in both good physical and mental health. Even simple stretching or going on a simple walk every day is better than doing nothing. Exercise can release endorphins which are hormones that help you feel better and this can help you feel more confident.

Practice positive affirmations – It might sound silly at first, but practice looking in the mirror every day and saying positive affirmations about yourself. Remind yourself of the things that you like and respect about yourself and every day repeat the fact that you are wonderful, worth loving, and a great person. Create a positive mantra for yourself and practice saying it at least twice a day.

Make an effort – Sometimes just making an effort to look good will make you feel good. It's easy to sit around the house all day in your housecoat and pajamas but try to make an effort to get dressed, brush your hair, and look good. You don't have to go anywhere or do anything huge, but taking care with your appearance lets your mind know that you still care about how you look on the outside. This might trick your body into start feeling better on the inside.

Stand straight – Your teacher and mother were both right when they told you to stand up straight. You don't have to carry a book on your head unless you want to, but do try to straighten your shoulders and your back. When you carry yourself well you'll feel more confident. Practice making eye contact and straightening your posture. Not only is it good for your back, it shows other people that you're confident and it will subliminally send the message that you're someone to treat with respect. When they start treating you with respect, you'll be more likely to treat yourself with respect.

Be thankful – When you're facing a chronic illness like CKD it's always easy to think about the things that are going wrong instead of the things that are going well for you. Every day, try to think of at least one thing that is going right in your life. Write it down if you have to. Be thankful and grateful for this. By trying to be positive about at least one thing it will help you create positive energy around you. This will do wonders for your confidence and keep you from sliding into totally negative thoughts.

Think of others –Take your mind off of your own issues and think of others. Volunteer at a local charity, even if you can't do it regularly.

Make healthy dietary choices – Work with your dietitian to make healthy eating choices. Pay careful attention to what you are consuming. A lot of heavy, processed foods can have effects on your mood. Fresh, whole foods can be better for your mental health. Get a meal plan or talk to your doctor about the kinds of foods that are good for both your physical and mental wellbeing.

Think positive- Think positive and give yourself time to sort out your feelings and your emotions before you react to anything. Use humor to lighten up the situation when you can.

Strategies to Help You Be More Positive

Use statements that are optimistic. Be encouraging and optimistic towards yourself. When you are pessimistic, you can unintentionally be using a self-fulfilling prophecy. Instead, be confident in your abilities to master even the most challenging of situations.

Be forgiving. Be as forgiving toward yourself as you would be toward someone you love. You won't always handle every aspect of your condition the way you think you should and that is okay.

Avoid using any statement that uses the word 'should.' Always use reasonable expectations with yourself or else you might be setting yourself up for failure. For instance, try to avoid telling yourself things like, "I *should* be able to run 2 miles without feeling tired" when that just might not be physically possible. Or, "I *should* be able to get through the day without having to stop for a small nap" when, in actuality, a small nap might actually give you the energy boost you need in order to feel revitalized. Since your limits can change, you don't want to place any on yourself that you simply can't live up to and that are impractical.

Look at your skills. Everyone has skills they have used that have gotten them through tough times in their lives. You are no different. Look at the skills you have and praise yourself for *these* skills.

Reframe negativity. When you find yourself thinking in a negative manner, reframe the negativity and use it as a learning tool. Address the negativity and understand that it's an indication that you should start reframing the situation in a new, more positive, way.

It is always going to be difficult to really love a body that sometimes doesn't seem to like you. Dealing with the symptoms and side effects of medications can get frustrating. It is important to learn to use strategies to deal with negative thoughts. Although you can't be positive all the time, since that is simply not realistic, learning to create a mostly positive energy around you will help make for a more pleasant atmosphere so that you can enjoy a better quality of life in general.

Medical Issues

There are several medical issues that can affect an individual and make them extremely uncomfortable, and even dangerously ill, when they are living with chronic kidney disease. Some of these issues will not only make it difficult to engage in sexual activity but may be the deciding factor in going ahead with dialysis, too.

Swelling/Edema

Swelling, or edema, is when the body fills with too much fluid or cannot remove excess fluid. Most people first notice this in their legs and face. It might start out as a puffiness but can later turn into a hard or firm to the touch area of the body. It can make walking and moving difficult and be very painful. Edema occurs either due to a loss of protein through the urine or impaired kidney function. Depending on the severity of the edema, it can be treated in a number of ways. There are medications that might be helpful in controlling it, for instance, like ACE inhibitors. Many individuals, however, need dialysis. If the swelling is too uncomfortable and painful then it might be difficult to for sexual activity to resume to a normal level until after the swelling has gone down.

Uremia

A build up of waste in the blood, called uremia, can oftentimes lead to nausea and vomiting. This can cause a general feeling of sickness that may or may not go away with time. Some individuals have trouble eating when this happens and also experience difficulty taking their medications since they aren't able to hold anything down. With this feeling of sickness, it can be hard to feel attractive, and even harder to feel like being involved with your partner in a sexual nature. As the stages of kidney failure progress, uremia worsens until dialysis starts.

Dehydration can also be a concern during this time, especially if you're unable to hold down any liquids. It's important that you talk to your doctor about any prolonged periods of vomiting. There are medications that might help with the vomiting. In extreme cases, an IV might be warranted in order to get hydration back into your system. In the meantime, practicing other forms of intimacy until you can be sexually active again can be a good way of staying close without engaging in intercourse.

Changes in Urination

Many people experience changes in urination, although not everyone experiences it in the same way. Some individuals notice that they have to urinate more frequently while others don't have to go as much. For some individuals, they have a pressing desire to urinate but, once they reach the restroom, can't empty their bladder completely. This can actually be very painful and result in multiple trips to the restroom for them.

In terms of sexuality, changes in urination can be embarrassing. It can be disruptive and worrisome for both partners. Learning to work around these disruptions might take some creative maneuvers and problem-solving techniques. It will also take come communication on the part of both partners.

If you experience any changes in your urination, including the color of your urine, it's important to talk to your doctor about what you are experiencing.

Male and Female Fertility

Both men and women with chronic kidney disease may face problems with infertility. Women, especially, might have difficulty becoming pregnant since they often experience disruptions in their menstrual cycles which can make it complicated to determine when they are ovulating. Some women also experience a stop in menstrual cycles altogether. Since more than 50% of men can have erectile dysfunction problems, they might also experience problems if they are trying to conceive as well. There have also been some demonstrated hormonal changes seen in individuals on dialysis. Increased levels of luteinizing hormone (LH) have been seen in men while the opposite has been reported in women. For women, this can be detrimental if they wish to become pregnant since the luteinizing hormone is needed for fertilization and is increased during times of ovulation. Low levels can cause missed periods and infertility. On the other hand, high levels of LH in men can cause testicular failure and also lead to fertility problems.

Chronic renal failure can negatively affect sperm quality and fertility and cause erection problems which can indirectly have an impact on fertility. If you are trying to conceive then it's important to talk to your doctor and your OBGYN about any issues you might be experiencing.

Pregnancy

In pregnancy, there is a high risk of miscarriage and an increased risk of difficulties for women with chronic kidney disease. Women with CKD have a risk of premature delivery and preeclampsia it's therefore important to work with a doctor who is familiar with CKD. The pregnancy itself would be considered high-risk in most cases.

There is a risk that the pregnancy can worsen the kidney function, or that decreased kidney function might interfere with the pregnancy.

However, this would be dependent upon several different factors. A woman, for instance, with mild to moderate chronic kidney disease who is thinking about becoming pregnant should discuss the possible risks with her nephrologist and obstetrical provider before conceiving to discuss these factors.

Those individuals with end-stage kidney disease who are on dialysis and become pregnant are at most risk and should consider their situation very closely before conceiving. They should also work very closely with their doctors. Some of their risk factors include being at very high risk for miscarriage, preeclampsia, premature delivery, and severe hypertension. However, an individual who has a successful renal transplantation has a lower risk of these complications. Therefore, it's important to consider the individual's complete history and extenuating factors before making any decisions based on one element.

Preeclampsia is one of the most dangerous conditions that can develop for both baby and mother during pregnancy and a complication that women with chronic kidney disease are at higher risk for, although women without CKD can still develop it. Preeclampsia normally causes high blood pressure and there can also be leak of protein from the kidneys into the urine. Although the majority of cases are mild, some are severe and necessitate early delivery of the baby.

Because kidney disease impedes hormones that usually regulate menstruation, a lot of women with kidney disease find their periods become irregular or stop altogether. It can therefore become complicated to identify pregnancy. Some women only infer that they are pregnant when they develop other inexplicable symptoms such as nausea.

If you become pregnant after a transplant then as long as the transplant is functioning well, you have the best chance of a normal pregnancy. If the transplant is not going well, then complications may arise, including the chances of deterioration in the transplant itself. It might be important to take anti-rejection therapy throughout pregnancy. If you want to become pregnant, this should be discussed with your medical team as soon as possible.

Communication

Communication is always important in any relationship but discussing any problems effectively with your partner is essential when you are dealing with both sexual issues and your problems surrounding your chronic kidney disease. Most problems that occur in the relationship are due to the fact that there is a breakdown in communication. Relationships can suffer when partners don't discuss their problems that have obvious solutions. The absence of discussions can lead to feelings of distance and lack of intimacy. It's important to find ways to talk candidly about the challenges you are facing. In fact, it's probably the first step toward successful problem-solving and the feelings of intimacy that come from a good partnership.

A lot of individuals with CKD end up feeling tired, worried, anxious, and frightened. All of these can diminish your energy inhibit your ability to demonstrate your affections toward your partner effectively. This can also affect your sexuality and cause a breakdown in communication.

Talking about and problems or issues you might be having and sharing your anxieties and fears will give you the chance to work through them and get the support you need. Although avoiding your problems might feel good at the time, it really is imperative to deal you're your emotions, even those that may seem despondent. In fact, some people find they actually feel better once they've dealt with some of the morbid fears they have, such as dying, because it gives them a sense of control and relief back into their lives. Sometimes, it's the feeling of not having any control that is the most overwhelming feeling. Making plans and setting small goals might be helpful, even if they seem morbid to others.

Of course, you don't want to talk about your problems all the time. If you're consumed with talking about your medical issues, and nothing else, then that's also a problem. And if you never talk about it, that's a problem. There has to be some sort of middle ground in order for the communication to be healthy.

If you do feel as though you need to talk to someone other than your partner, then you should speak to your physician because they can refer you to a clinical psychology service. A counselor can often be a good neutral outside listener because, while a partner can offer support, you might feel as though you need to talk to someone else from time to time.

Knowing Where To Start

Sometimes it's difficult to tell whether sexual problems are due to physical or emotional causes. You should work with your doctor to determine what might be causing any sexual problems you might be experiencing. A complete medical, psychological and sexual history of you might be required. One of the first things your doctor might do is review your medications and their side effects since these often cause sexual dysfunctions. Blood tests should include hormone levels and blood sugar levels to check for diabetes. Men can be checked to see if nerve and blood supply to the penis are good and if they can have an erection. A sexual history of both you and your partner might be considered as well. If no physical problem is found, an emotional cause must be considered.

Talking to your partner, and even your doctor, about your sexuality can be difficult. Even in modern times, it can be embarrassing to discuss something so intimate. Still, keep in mind that your sexuality is an important part of your total well-being, just like the rest of your health. Although it can be difficult to talk about it and you may be embarrassed to discuss your sexual feelings or performance, your doctors are trained to help you with any medical issues you may be experiencing, just as they are trained to help you with any issues you have regarding your kidneys.

Talking about sex can be difficult. When you're talking with your partner:

1. Think about what you're going to say before you say it
2. Pick a time to talk when you're both relaxed and can concentrate.
3. Don't discuss it after a trying day.
4. Select a place where you both feel comfortable.
5. Don't make up excuses.
6. Don't blame your partner for anything.
7. Let your partner share their feelings and listen to what they're saying.
8. Don't try to guess at what one another is trying to say. Let each other finish the other's thoughts.

Working Through Issues

When the problems are emotional and not physical, the treatment options usually include some form of counseling. Emotional issues might include, but are not limited to, one of the following:

Grief: Being diagnosed with a chronic illness, especially in the beginning, does often send many people into the grief cycle. As a result, some people do end up experiencing the stages of grief which can include depression. As a result, a lack of interest in sexual activity can form due to a chemical imbalance triggered by the depression.

Fear of rejection or failed performance: A fear of rejection or failed performance is very common after surgery or when there has been a significant change in a person's body. You might, for instance, no longer feel "whole" or "complete" and worry that you'll no longer be able to perform like you were once able to. This might result in a loss of confidence. A change in the way your body looks might also cause a lack of self-esteem.

Anxiety: Worries about your future, your health, and even mounting medical bills can all take precedent in your mind and make it difficult to become sexually aroused and focus on sexual activity. This can make it difficult to become aroused at all or to achieve orgasm.

Guilt: Ironically, sometimes guilt at not being sexually active in the past can become so strong that it can make it difficult to perform in the present. It can place too much pressure to perform in the present and the body is unable to respond to the stress. Other times, the mind may worry that you're overexerting yourself or worry that you should be doing something "more important" and make it difficult for you to become aroused. A partner might feel guilty and worry that they are going to hurt their loved one who might have recently gotten a transplant or had dialysis and the guilt might make it difficult for them to become aroused, for instance.

Changes in family roles: Sometimes, the traditional family roles may become reversed and this could have an effect on the sexual roles in the family as well. If the male, for example, has always been the breadwinner but suddenly becomes disabled and is no longer able to work then he might feel guilty and emasculated that his wife is now employed and paying the bills. This could have an effect on his sexual performance. Working with a counselor in these situations will often provide the best solutions.

Relationships and Social Changes

Restless nights, dialysis routine, dietary and fluid restrictions, and fatigue can all necessitate lifestyle adjustments. Although practical, these changes can eventually put heavy strains on all your personal relationships, but especially affect your everyday relationship with your partner when it comes to intimacy.

A noteworthy consideration for you and your partner to consider is that of dialysis. The treatment may take up a lot of time which may eat up into time that you would normally spend together, doing things that you enjoy. This might mean that you no longer have the free time to go out and socialize that you used to. Some couples find it frustrating that they can't relax and enjoying themselves in the way they're used to. As a result, conflicts might arise as they attempt to adjust into new routines.

It's also easy to fall into a new routine where sex is just too easy to ignore and avoid because it's too much work, especially if fatigue is a problem or you don't have the extra time to fit it in. This is common if you are now sleeping in different rooms due to restlessness or different sleeping patterns. It's important to try to maintain intimacy, even if the situation becomes complicated, since intimacy is a big part of any relationship. This might mean making a special effort to ensure that you make one-on-one time for your relationship.

How to Bring It Up

It's never easy bringing up the fact that you have a chronic condition but how do you let someone know that you have chronic kidney disease, especially if you're considering entering into a relationship with them? The following is a quick guide of suggestions to keep in mind when you're having the first conversation with them and tips that you might want to consider.

1. **Determine if you need to tell them.** You don't have to tell everyone you meet that you have CKD. Of course, you can if you want to, but if it makes you uncomfortable then don't share the news unless you have to. Think about your reasons for telling them. If you have just met them for the first time and it's a casual date and you're not "clicking" then you might not be planning on seeing them again. There may not

be a reason to share your diagnosis. However, if you feel like future dates are in order and the relationship could become more serious then it's a conversation that is probably worth having.

2. **Consider your timing.** Your chronic kidney disease is a serious subject. You want to bring it up when you have your date's attention. But you also don't want to ruin the mood which can make the rest of the evening or afternoon awkward and uncomfortable. Consider bringing up the subject during a conversation when you're talking about other important topics and not, for instance, right before the movie starts, or during a lighthearted moment. You want to give your partner time to process the information.

3. **Consider the place.** As well as considering the timing, consider the place that you have the conversation in as well. A quiet place where you can talk is ideal. A noisy, crowded restaurant where you can barely hear one another is *not* ideal. A group date where other people are around is not a private moment and might put your date, and you, on the spot.

4. **Make it personal.** Writing it out in a text or email might make it easier on you but it's far less personal. In this digital day and age, some things are still better said in person. Your partner, or potential partner, may have a lot of questions for you regarding your CKD. It's probably better that you're there to answer them instead of going back and forth through the computer or phone. Things can get lost in digital translation.

5. **Keep it simple.** Try to keep your explanations as simple as possible. You probably know a lot about CKD. Your partner may not be as interested in all of the medical terminology as you are. What they may be interested in, however, are any limitations you have and what kind of prognosis you have. Be prepared for these kinds of questions. Keep your

emphasis on how well you're doing, the kind of support you have, and what you're looking for (and not looking for).

6. **Don't give away too much.** Your health problems are ultimately your own. You don't have to give any details that you don't feel comfortable talking about.

7. **Be prepared for a change of subject.** Some people simply don't know what to say. They need time to process the information they've been given. Don't be surprised if you tell your potential partner, or partner, about your diagnosis and you get a very underwhelming response and a change of subject. This doesn't necessarily mean that they're not interested in you and your health. It could simply mean that they need some time to think about what you just told them. You might return home later and find a message from them with lots of questions. Or, you could get that message a week later.

8. **Be prepared.** If they do want more information try to have some brochures or websites that you can point them in the direction of.

9. **But don't be pushy.** If they act disinterested, however, don't force these brochures or websites on them. Some people like to find this information on their own and will do their own searching and investigating. Simply let them know that the information is out there and exists.

10. **Relax.** Once you've shared your news, try to relax and have fun. You might feel as though a weight has been lifted off your shoulders. Sharing the news of your CKD will at least allow you to be honest in your new relationship and permit you to move forward, one way or another.

11. **If You Are In A Relationship.** Discuss intimacy and your fears with your significant other. Talk about how you feel about the changes in your relationship with regards to the role changes in your family. Now that you are possibly more reliant on them, your relationship has changed and it may

make your intimate relationship different. If you talk about it, it can be easier to address, especially if you talk about it before you start to have an issue.

Seeking Help

It *is* possible to get help to work out sexual issues. Don't be afraid or uncomfortable to ask your doctor, counselor, or social worker for help. Therapy can focus on such things as improving communication and increasing awareness of how the person with chronic kidney disease feels. Sharing individual sexual needs and difficulties with a partner can generate understanding and even more intimacy. Learning new coping skills are also important in resuming a healthy sex. If medication is an issue then your doctor might also be able to help as well by changing medication if possible.

Sex Therapy

Sex therapy has been helpful for some couples as they learn new ways to connect with their partners in different physical manners. In sex therapy, sexual problems are dealt with for both partners and individuals. Sexual education is administered and the therapist also assigns activities as homework which include stress reduction activities, communication exercises, and giving and receiving pleasurable touches.

Some of the different issues that sex therapy can help with include a lack of interest in sexual activity, trouble reaching orgasm, and pain during intercourse. For individuals with CKD, sex therapy can help individuals work through the effects of chronic illness on sexuality.

Sex therapists can be psychiatrists, psychologist, doctors, and social workers. They should be licensed and have advanced training and experience in sexuality and sexual issues. Your insurance might even cover at least some of your visits to the therapist.

Counseling

Sometimes regular counseling, either couples therapy or alone, can be helpful when it comes to sorting out feelings around sexuality. Talking about emotional issues and body issues can be useful in dealing with depression and anxiety. Your partner should be supportive but professional help is important to get when you're dealing with complicated issues that you need extra assistance with. Sometimes, your partner might want to attend sessions with you as well. You might find that counseling can help you not only in your sexual issues but in other aspects of your life as well, especially if you are having trouble sleeping or digestive problems.

Don't forget that there are online forums and groups to consider if you aren't comfortable talking to a local person face-to-face at first. You can find answers sometimes without posting a thing.

Treatments

For men with erectile dysfunctions, there are quite a few options available that might be appropriate depending on what is causing the issue. For instance, it's possible for inflatable or semi-rigid rods to be inserted into the penis via surgery in extreme cases. Surgery has also been shown to help improve the penis' blood flow, too, which can help erectile dysfunction. Male hormones may be administered if surgery isn't desired. Specially trained doctors who are skilled in impotence can offer information on all available options to those who are having trouble with erectile dysfunction so it's essential to talk to your physician about any difficulty you may be having so that you can find the best treatment that is most suited to you and your condition. Help most likely is available so it's important to communicate with your medical team.

For women experiencing vaginal dryness, and those who have low hormone levels, a water-soluble vaginal lubricant might be able to significantly decrease or stop intercourse pain. In addition, those women who are unable to reach orgasm or may need additional time to become aroused due to fatigue, hormone changes, or medications might need a change in medication or extra hormones. If you feel like any of these issues might apply to you then these are things that you should bring up to your doctor. Sometimes, the answer can be as simple as a change in medication or an over-the-counter product that can be used each time you have intercourse. Your doctor should be able to give you more information about any choices that are available to you.

How Patients Can Help Themselves

It's important to learn to stand up for yourself and help yourself when you can.

- **Be your own advocate**: you're always going to be your own best advocate when it comes to your health.

- **Limit alcohol**: alcohol can intensify the symptoms of anxiety and depression and adversely interact with some medications.

- **Stop smoking**: smoking can cause further damage to your issues and could aggravate other sexual problems that you might be experiencing.

- **Learn stress management techniques**: stress management techniques, such as meditation or journaling, can help with symptoms of anxiety and depression.

- **Practice good communication skills**: practice good communication skills with their partners in order to foster a healthy atmosphere within their relationships to ensure that their needs are being met.

- **Attend counseling**: if you find that you need additional help, attend counseling sessions with either a traditional psychiatrist or psychologist or a sex therapist so that you can work on sexual dysfunctions that might be causing you issues.

Boosting Your Self-Esteem

There are additional ways that might help increase your self-confidence and boost your self-esteem while you continue to work with your doctors and your partner on your needs. Just remember to keep the lines of communication open at all times and don't neglect to focus on being your own best advocate for the things you need.

- Take as much time as you can with your personal grooming. When you look good, you tend to feel good.
- Do your best not to think of sexual intercourse as the only kind of sexual act since this may cause you unnecessary frustration if you are currently experiencing limited sexual desire or energy.
- If you feel awkward talking about sex with others, books and online resources can be a good forms of self-help. Visit your library or bookstore and find a book that deals with your issues or search online. The anonymity might help ease your shyness until you feel more confident talking to your doctor.
- Focus on making small goals and sticking to them. Feel proud of small accomplishments and give yourself credit when you do something you set out to do.
- Don't hold yourself up to past achievements. It's easy to lose confidence in your sexuality when you consider the way you were in the past but, instead, focus on what you can do in the present and in the future.

More Than Sex

There are lots of ways to communicate intimacy and please each other without going through with actual intercourse. You can experience intimacy and still convey desire, intimacy, devotion, and fondness for one another. Here are a few simple suggestions other than intercourse:

- Make special time for each other.

- Go to doctors' visits together.

- Stay aware of what's going on in each others' lives.

- Allow your partner to have a break from your treatments.

- Seek professional help from counselors and therapists.

- Maintain interests that are separate from your partner's.

- Maintain interests that are shared with your partner.

- Do at least one thing together every week that doesn't include anyone else.

- Have conversations that don't revolve around your medical treatment or your family life.

As most happy couples will tell you, while nobody can let you in on the clue to keeping up a contented relationship when one partner has chronic kidney disease and the other doesn't, you *can* be honest with each other and support each other's needs. When you respect and trust one another you're more apt to endure the difficult times and take pleasure in the good ones together.

If you've just started a new relationship you may have qualms about yourself and feel less attractive. You might even be going through some changes in your lifestyle, such as dietary restrictions or dialysis demands, and have apprehension due to sexual issues and body changes. Just keep in mind that we're usually more judgmental of ourselves than others are, though.

If you aren't in a relationship, before you decide to get involved with someone, you might want to determine if you have the energy to give a significant other. Some of this decision will be based on how you are feeling. Consider how you're feeling, how much energy you have, how much time you have to devote to someone at the moment.

It can be hard to tell a prospective partner or new relationship about any sexual or fertility issues since this is a very sensitive and personal subject. Still, it's important that you're honest with them as soon as possible.

Conclusion

Your sexuality doesn't have to end with your diagnosis of chronic kidney disease. It is possible to maintain a healthy, active sex life and to continue feeling good about your sexuality, your body image, and yourself. It's always important to remember that you are not alone in your journey and, when in doubt, your doctors and social worker, if you have one, should be able to point you in the direction of support groups of others who might be dealing with the same issues.

There aren't any limits in regards to sexual activities you may engage in with your partner as someone with renal disease, just as long as the activity doesn't place any pressure or tension on the access site which could potentially cause damage. Still, if you are sexually active, it's important to practice safe sex unless you're in a committed relationship and to use birth control or else discuss pregnancy options with your medical team.

If you are unable to engage in intercourse for different reasons, there are other ways to enjoy intimacy. Other enjoyable activities such as kissing, touching, and hugging offer partners feelings of closeness and intimacy even when actual intercourse isn't involved.

One of the best things you can do is keep an open mind about your situation and maintain a positive attitude about yourself and your sexuality. This might be difficult at times, but it may actually lower your chances of having additional sexual issues. It can also help you in other areas of your life, too, and a positive attitude has been shown to have positive effects on overall health.

Certain relaxation techniques and stress relieving activities might be helpful in relieving tension and anxiety. Journaling, meditation, blogging, and even exercising are all ways of working out tension and channeling frustration and stress in positive outlets. Support group sessions might help you connect with others who are going through similar situations with intimate counseling sessions might offer you the one-on-one support you need from a professional. A therapist might help you feel better about your body image and/or sexual dysfunction that you might be experiencing.

If you are experiencing any other problems that can be attributed to your chronic kidney disease then resuming previous pleasurable activities, such as dining out or traveling, as a couple, can be helpful in relieving any stress you might be feeling.

Lastly, don't forget to communicate with your partner about how you feel. It's easy to assume that those around you know and understand your feelings but unless you take the time to verbalize them there's a very real possibility that they simply have no idea what you are experiencing or going through. Many problems couples face are due to lack of communication.

Life *can* be good again and will be!

Other Titles By Mathea Ford:

Mathea Ford, Author Page (all books):

http://www.amazon.com/Mathea-Ford/e/B008E1E7IS/

The Kidney Friendly Diet Cookbook

http://www.amazon.com/Kidney-Friendly-Diet-Cookbook-PreDialysis-ebook/dp/B00BC7BGPI/

Create Your Own Kidney Diet Plan

http://www.amazon.com/Create-Your-Kidney-Diet-Plan-ebook/dp/B009PSN3R0/

Living with Chronic Kidney Disease - Pre-Dialysis

http://www.amazon.com/Living-Chronic-Kidney-Disease-Pre-Dialysis-ebook/dp/B008D8RSAQ/

Eating a Pre-Dialysis Kidney Diet - Calories, Carbohydrates, Fat & Protein, Secrets To Avoid Dialysis

http://www.amazon.com/Eating-Pre-Dialysis-Kidney-Diet-Carbohydrates-ebook/dp/B00DU2JCHM/

Eating a Pre-Dialysis Kidney Diet - Sodium, Potassium, Phosphorus and Fluids, A Kidney Disease Solution

http://www.amazon.com/Eating-Pre-Dialysis-Kidney-Diet-Phosphorus-ebook/dp/B00E2U8VMS/

Eating Out On a Kidney Diet: Pre-dialysis and Diabetes: Ways To Enjoy Your Favorite Foods

http://www.amazon.com/Eating-Out-Kidney-Diet-Pre-dialysis/dp/0615928781/

Kidney Disease: Common Labs and Medical Terminology: The Patient's Perspective

http://www.amazon.com/Kidney-Disease-Terminology-Perspective-Pre-Dialysis/dp/0615931804/

Dialysis: Treatment Options for the Progression to End Stage Renal Disease

http://www.amazon.com/Dialysis-Treatment-Options-Progression-Disease/dp/0615932258/

Mindful Eating For A Pre-Dialysis Kidney Diet: Healthy Attitudes Toward Food and Life

http://www.amazon.com/Mindful-Eating-Pre-Dialysis-Kidney-Diet/dp/0615933475/

The Emotional Challenges Of Coping with Chronic Kidney Disease

http://www.amazon.com/Emotional-Challenges-Chronic-Disease-Dialysis-ebook/dp/B00H6SYQG8/

Heart Healthy Living with Kidney Disease: Lowering Blood Pressure

http://www.amazon.com/Heart-Healthy-Living-Kidney-Disease/dp/0615936059/

Exercising with Chronic Kidney Disease: Solutions To An Active Lifestyle

http://www.amazon.com/Exercising-Chronic-Kidney-Disease-Solutions/dp/0615936342/

Sign up for our email list to learn of new titles right away!

http://www.renaldiethq.com/go/email/